Sciatica Exercises & Home Treatment

Simple, Effective Care For Sciatica And Piriformis Syndrome

By Dr. George Best, D.C.

Sciatica Exercises & Home Treatment

Copyright © 2012 George F. Best, D.C.. All Rights Reserved.

ISBN-13: 978-1494743765

[Type text]

Table Of Contents

Disclaimer 1
Chapter 1: Understanding Sciatica 2
   Basic Spinal Anatomy 2
   Disc Protrusion / Bulge / Herniation 3
   Disc Extrusion / Rupture 4
   Degenerative Bone and Ligament Thickening 5
   Sciatic Nerve and Piriformis Muscle 6
Chapter 2: Discovering The Cause Of Your Sciatica 8
   Clue #1 - Posture 8
   Clue #2 – Standing Up After Prolonged Sitting 9
   Clue #3 – Symptoms Associated With Heavy Lifting / Repeated Bending 9
   Clue #4 – Sciatica That Develops After Inactivity 10
   Clue #5 – Reaction to Applying Heat 10
   Clue #6 – The Straight-Leg Test 10
   Clue #7 – The Piriformis Stretch Test 11
   Interpreting the Clues 12
Chapter 3: Relieving Symptoms With Ice And Heat 14
Chapter 4: Sciatica Symptom Relief Exercises 16
   McKenzie Method Exercises 18
      Advanced McKenzie Extension Technique 21
      Modified McKenzie Extension Technique 23
   Exercises for Muscle Contraction Sciatica 23
      Piriformis Stretching 24
      Gluteus Minimus Stretching 25
Chapter 5: Massage And Positioning Techniques 26
   Self-Massage 26
      Piriformis Massage 26
      Gluteus Minimus Massage 27
   Pelvic Repositioning 28
   Enhancing Sitting Comfort 29
Chapter 6: Acupressure Techniques 31
   Pen Button and Laser Methods Of Acupressure Stimulation 31
   Point GB34 For General Musculoskeletal Pain 32
   Sciatica Points 32
   Low Back Pain Points 33
   Auriculotherapy (Ear Acupressure) Points 34
   "Surround the Dragon" 34
Chapter 7: Supplements And Natural Remedies 36

    Natural Anti-Inflammatories 36
    Correcting Nutrient Deficiencies 37
Chapter 8: Releasing Emotional Pain Triggers 40
    Points for Emotional Freedom Technique 41
Chapter 9: Prevention Of Sciatica 44
    The Importance of Prevention 44
    Back Safe Posture and Lifting 45
        Poor Sitting Posture 45
        Good Sitting Posture 46
        Sleep Position 46
        Bending and Lifting 47
        Poor Bending, Lifting, and Carrying 47
        Safer Bending, Lifting, and Carrying 48
    Preventive Exercises 48
        The Pelvic Tilt 49
        The Slouch and Arch 51
    Preventive Exercise Summary 51
Chapter 10: When To See A Doctor 53
    Cauda Equina Syndrome 53
    Failure to Improve Within 2 to 3 Weeks 53
    Pain Becoming Numbness 54
Conclusion 55
About The Author 56
Review And Connect 57

Disclaimer

Every case is different and although the vast majority of sciatica sufferers will improve using the treatment methods presented, this book is not a substitute for professional evaluation and treatment. Some individuals may require different or additional treatments to the ones presented in this book. Readers are advised to pay close attention to the warnings and precautions that are included in this book and are advised to seek medical attention in the event that symptoms worsen or if new symptoms arise.

If you have questions or would like additional information, please visit the author's website, www.SciaticaTreatmentAtHome.com, or email the author at info@sciaticaselfcare.com.

Chapter 1: Understanding Sciatica

The term sciatica refers to symptoms arising from the sciatic nerve, which is the large nerve formed from several smaller nerves that branch off from each side of the lower spine. The sciatic nerves pass through the buttock area on each side and then continue down the back of each leg. Below the knee, the sciatic nerve splits into two divisions that continue down the leg to the ankle and foot.

Although some people call symptoms anywhere in the leg sciatica, true sciatica symptoms occur in the buttock area and may extend down the back of the thigh and into the lower leg and foot. Generally, the more irritated the nerve is, the further the symptoms will extend down the leg.

While there are rare neurological disorders that can cause the development of sciatica due to direct nerve pathology, in most cases sciatica is a symptom of some other underlying problem. The most common causes of sciatica can be broken down into two main categories, nerve compression and muscle contraction.

Nerve compression can result from a variety of causes, but it is most commonly caused by a bulge or rupture of one or more intervertebral discs in the lower lumbar spine. The illustration below shows the basic anatomy of a section of the spine as viewed from the side:

Basic Spinal Anatomy

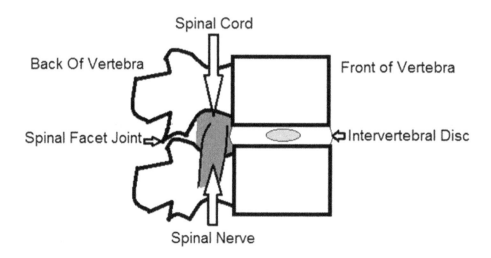

Under normal circumstances, there is plenty of space around the spinal nerves where they branch off from the spinal cord and exit the spine (technically, the spinal cord ends in the mid lumbar spine and becomes a bundle of separate nerves called the cauda equina in the lower lumbars, but for the sake of simplicity, I'll be referring to it as the spinal cord). But the opening where the nerve exits the spine can become narrowed by one or more things, resulting in compression and irritation of the nerve.

One of the most common sources of nerve compression is a disc bulge, which is also known as a disc herniation, or disc protrusion. The discs have an outer cartilage wall and are filled with a gel-like material that provides the spine with multiple angles of mobility and shock-absorption. The wall can become damaged (in ways that will be discussed later) and the inner pressure of the gel causes it to bulge outward at the point of damage. Because of the structure of the spine, and because of the postures and activities that we commonly engage in, discs tend to bulge backwards towards the spinal cord and nerves. This is illustrated below:

Disc Protrusion / Bulge / Herniation

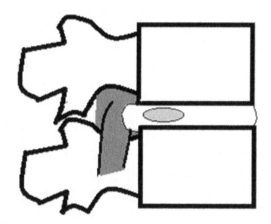

In severe cases of disc damage, the disc may actually rupture, and the inner gel will actually come through the disc wall. This is called a disc rupture or disc extrusion and is shown on the next page:

Disc Extrusion / Rupture

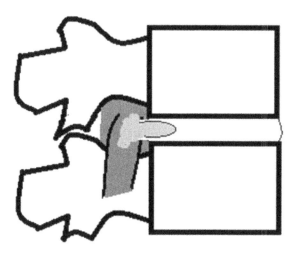

The vast majority of disc injuries are bulges or protrusions and can usually be effectively treated with the methods that will be discussed later in this book. Disc ruptures (extrusions) are more serious and will often require surgery to achieve long-term relief of symptoms. By the way, the term "ruptured disc" frequently gets used incorrectly (even by doctors) to describe what is actually a disc bulge (herniation or protrusion), so don't assume that you will need surgery if you are told you have a ruptured disc until you have confirmation (from an MRI or CT scan) that the disc is in fact ruptured (the terms "extruded" or "sequestered" will appear on the imaging reports in reference to one or more discs) and not simply bulging or protruding.

In addition to disc bulges and ruptures, the space around the spinal nerves are commonly narrowed by changes in the spine related to degenerative arthritis. With degenerative arthritis, the discs will often lose fluid and become thinner, bone surfaces may thicken and/or form spurs, and spinal ligaments may buckle (from the bones becoming closer together) and/or become thicker – all of which may narrow the openings the nerves pass through. These types of changes are illustrated on the next page:

Degenerative Bone and Ligament Thickening

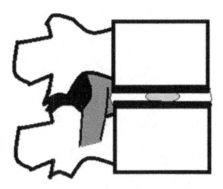

Degenerative changes in the spine most often affect the back part of the spinal openings, while disc bulges and ruptures usually narrow the front side of the spinal openings. In many cases, there is some degree of narrowing from both disc protrusion and degenerative changes. In addition, further nerve compression often results from swelling due to inflammation that is triggered by disc damage and/or degenerative arthritis.

While nerve compression can also result from tumors and spinal cysts which require surgical treatment, the majority of cases of nerve compression are due to some combination of disc bulging, degenerative changes, and/or inflammatory swelling and can usually be effectively managed with the treatments discussed later in this book.

The other major category of causes of sciatica symptoms is muscle contraction. Several muscles can cause pain down the leg, but only one muscle really matches the symptoms of true sciatic nerve irritation. The piriformis is a muscle located in the lower buttock area on each side that attaches from the sacrum (the triangular bone at the base of the spine) to the upper femur, just below the hip joint. The right piriformis muscle is shown in the picture that follows:

Sciatic Nerve and Piriformis Muscle

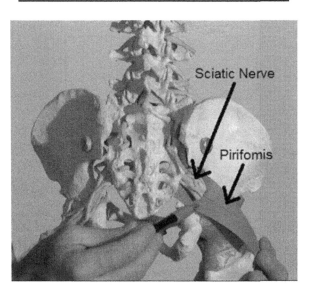

Anatomy varies somewhat from person to person, and the sciatic nerve can pass above, below, or right through the piriformis muscle. It is believed that in cases where the nerve passes through the piriformis, contraction or tightness of the muscle can be sufficient to cause pressure irritation on the sciatic nerve, but it also appears that the muscle itself can produce referred pain symptoms that closely mimic the symptom pattern of sciatic nerve irritation. In any event, when the piriformis is associated with sciatic nerve symptoms, it is called "piriformis syndrome".

Piriformis syndrome can be brought on by direct trauma to the muscle, such as from a fall on the buttocks, but oftentimes arises simply after prolonged periods of sitting. Most cases of piriformis syndrome can be successfully treated with the techniques that are presented later in this book, but occasionally injections or even surgical treatment may be needed to reduce pressure on the sciatic nerve when it passes through the center of the muscle.

It should be noted that a given person can be suffering from piriformis syndrome as well as nerve compression at the spine at the same time. In fact, because the piriformis muscle is controlled by some of the same nerve components that form the sciatic nerve, disc bulges and other sources of compression can irritate those nerve components and that irritation in turn can cause the piriformis muscle to become excessively contracted and begin to produce symptoms of its own. Because of this, some have concluded that ALL cases of sciatica are related to piriformis contraction, but in my 20 plus years of clinical experience, I have not found this to be true.

As mentioned previously, there are other muscles that can produce symptoms similar to sciatica, although usually there are distinct differences in the symptom pattern. Sciatica symptoms due to nerve compression or from piriformis syndrome are typically in the buttock and down the back of the thigh, and sometimes into the lower leg and foot. Symptoms in the side or front of the thigh are not usually due to sciatica nor piriformis syndrome and involve other nerves, muscles, and/or other anatomical structures. Since the possible causes of non-sciatic leg symptoms are numerous, this book will be focusing primarily on treatment for true sciatica and piriformis syndrome.

As you may imagine, because the causes of sciatica vary, the most effective treatment methods will also vary from case to case. So, the first step in treating your sciatica is to try to figure out the most likely cause(s) of it and then apply the most appropriate treatments for your particular situation.

In the next chapter you'll learn ways to help determine the cause(s) of your sciatica.

Chapter 2: Discovering The Cause Of Your Sciatica

As was discussed in Chapter 1, there are several possible causes of sciatica, but most cases fall into one of two main categories: nerve compression and muscle contraction.

In some cases it may not be possible to determine 100% what the problem is without going through advanced medical testing (MRI, nerve conduction testing, etc.), and in a few cases even advanced testing is not completely reliable, but the procedures that follow should help give at least some idea of the likely causes of your symptoms.

As we go through the following clues to the causes of your sciatica, bear in mind that no indicator is a "stand alone". That is, you're looking for a general pattern among the various indicators discussed. For example, if out of the 7 clues, 4 suggest that your condition is due to nerve compression and 3 are inconclusive, assume that the problem is due to nerve compression.

Clue #1 - Posture

While not always present, sciatica due to nerve compression caused by a bulging disc will often be associated with a sideways shift of the upper body over the pelvis as shown in the picture below:

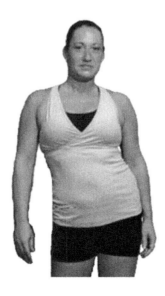

This type of postural shift is an unconscious protective mechanism the body has employed to reduce pressure on the damaged disc. There may or may not be low back pain present in addition to the sciatica symptoms. If you do have this type of sideways shift, it is best to NOT try to force yourself straight, as this will often dramatically increase symptoms. As your condition improves, your posture will gradually return to normal on its own.

Clue #2 – Standing Up After Prolonged Sitting

While prolonged sitting can lead to symptoms from both nerve compression due to disc bulging and from piriformis syndrome, when a disc is involved, there will usually be increased pain when initially trying to stand up straight, while in piriformis syndrome, standing upright does not usually make a big difference in symptoms.

Clue #3 – Symptoms Associated With Heavy Lifting / Repeated Bending

In most cases, sciatica that develops within one or two days after doing a lot of heavy lifting or repeated bending at the waist (such as with pulling weeds) is related to disc bulging. While most people have heard the advice to "lift with your legs", they may not understand the importance of this advice. When you bend forward at the waist, the mechanical stresses on the spinal discs tend to shift the pressure inside the discs backwards as indicated in the following illustration:

Shifts In Disc Pressure With Forward Bending

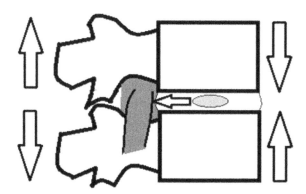

As the spine bends forward, there is compression at the front of the disc and a decompression at the back of the disc. This in turn causes the gel inside the disc to shift backwards towards the nerves.

If you bend forward frequently or if you are bending forward as you lift something heavy, this places strain on the back of the disc wall which can tear or overstretch it, leading to a disc bulge, or in extreme cases, a rupture.

Clue #4 – Sciatica That Develops After Inactivity

Whereas disc-related sciatica is associated with bending and lifting, sciatica from the piriformis muscle is often associated with inactivity. In particular sitting for long periods of time without getting up to move around, especially in a person who is usually more active, can lead to tightening of the piriformis.

Clue #5 – Reaction to Applying Heat

A common treatment for any type of musculoskeletal pain is to apply a heating pad or soak in a hot tub. In the case of nerve compression sciatica from a disc bulge or spinal degeneration, heat may feel good while it is being applied, but will usually increase inflammation and make symptoms worse overall in between applications. On the other hand, muscle contraction is usually eased by the application of heat, so piriformis syndrome and similar conditions will usually improve with the use of heat.

Clue #6 – The Straight-Leg Test

The straight-leg test checks for what doctors call "nerve root tension", which is a sign of nerve compression and irritation. To perform the test, simply sit up straight in a firm chair and straighten your leg at the knee as shown in the next image:

The Straight Leg Test

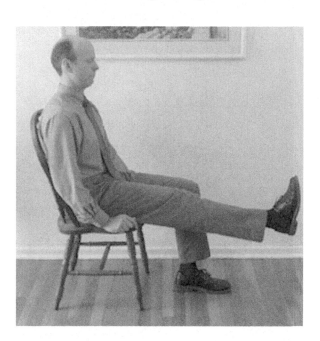

Do this test with both legs, even if you only have symptoms in one of them. An increase in pain in the symptomatic leg when straightening either leg is an indicator that you have nerve compression occurring, most often from a bulging disc. In the case of piriformis syndrome, the symptoms will usually either be unchanged or may even decrease during the straight-leg test.

Clue #7 – The Piriformis Stretch Test

The piriformis stretch test is basically what the name suggests, a stretch of the piriformis muscle. To do the test, slowly pull your knee towards the opposite-side shoulder as shown in the next picture:

The Piriformis Stretch Test

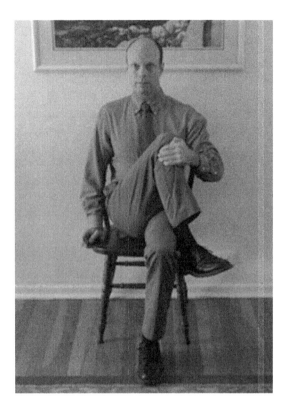

Increased pain in the buttock and/or leg is an indicator of piriformis tightness, but be sure to test the non-symptomatic leg as well. If there are increased symptoms in the non-symptomatic leg that are essentially the same as in the symptomatic leg, it could be due to overall inflammation and is not a reliable indicator of piriformis syndrome. Note that the increased pain may be short-lived, as the test does stretch the piriformis and is a treatment for piriformis syndrome as well as a test.

Interpreting the Clues

As mentioned at the beginning of this chapter, no one indicator by itself is reliable. Out of the 7 clues, you are looking for the majority of them to be in agreement as to the likely cause of your symptoms.

In the event that you don't get a clear indication as to the likely cause of your problem, I recommend assuming that the problem is nerve compression until proven otherwise by professional evaluation. This is because the treatments for muscle contraction have the potential to increase nerve compression symptoms. Although you may not get much better using the nerve compression treatments when you have a muscle contraction problem, it is unlikely that you would make the muscle contraction problem worse. So, when in doubt, always begin with the treatments for nerve compression.

Remember, it is entirely possible that you may have symptoms from both nerve compression and muscle contraction. In that case, for the reasons just discussed, always begin with the treatments for nerve compression and begin the treatments for piriformis syndrome (muscle contraction) later once the worst of the symptoms have eased.

With that in mind, let's proceed to the next chapter to discuss treatments to begin relieving your pain.

Chapter 3: Relieving Symptoms With Ice And Heat

One of the common confusions people have with self-treatment is the question of when to use ice and when to use heat. As we discussed in the previous chapter, ice is preferable when the issue is one of nerve compression, while heat is more effective for sciatica due to muscle contraction. In the last chapter we discussed various clues to determining the cause of your symptoms, but when in doubt, a simple rule of thumb is to base the decision of whether to use ice or heat on what the symptoms are.

If you have sharp or intense pain with or without swelling, this usually indicates that there is inflammation present, and this is a time to use ice. On the other hand, if your symptoms are mostly stiffness or mild soreness, there is usually not significant inflammation present, and in this situation heat is a better choice.

As a precaution, anytime you have experienced a trauma, or think you might have injured yourself, it is best to avoid using heat for at least 48 hours to make sure that the inflammatory response has not been activated and the inflammation has simply not had enough time to set in.

When in doubt, avoid using heat!

Although heat may feel good while it is on (because heat increases transmission of certain nerve signals that cause pain signals to be partially blocked from reaching the brain), heat also increases the inflammatory response of the body. Increased inflammation means increased pain when you stop using the heat.

Although ice may not feel as comfortable as heat, it is one of the best anti-inflammatory measures you can take. The short-term discomfort of applying ice usually pays off in long-term relief.

Although some experts recommend alternating ice and heat (for example, 10 minutes of ice followed by 10 minutes of heat), I have not seen any particular advantage in doing this. For most situations, choosing one or the other based on the symptoms as was just discussed is usually the simplest approach and in my experience works just as well or possibly better than trying to alternate the therapies.

Regardless of whether you are using ice or heat, you should always separate the ice or hot pack from the skin with a layer of cloth to prevent skin damage. It is also important to avoid applying ice or heat on an area that has been recently treated with Theragesic, Icy Hot, Biofreeze, Ben Gay, or any other topical analgesic - wait until the sensation of the analgesic has completely worn off, otherwise the ice or heat could cause skin irritation or damage.

Also when using either ice or heat, you should only apply the treatment for about 15 minutes at a time, allowing the skin to return to normal temperature (to be safe, allow 1 to 2 hours) before re-applying the treatment. As it may take a few minutes for the cold or warm sensation to make it through the cloth layer between the cold/hot pack and your skin, begin timing when you start to feel the temperature change on the skin.

IMPORTANT NOTE*: If you have impaired circulation or decreased skin sensitivity due to nerve damage, diabetes, etc., it is best to check with your doctor first before using ice or heat.

Chapter 4: Sciatica Symptom Relief Exercises

There are many exercises that have been suggested for the self-treatment of sciatica. I often come across people who have been given long, complicated lists of exercises by doctors or physical therapists. Most of these exercises are of minimal benefit at best and because of the complexity of the exercise regimen, most patients don't use them for very long.

In my 20 plus years of clinical experience, I have found that using just a few particularly effective exercises on a frequent basis is far more beneficial than having patients do a lot of different exercises.

In this chapter, I'll be presenting exercise recommendations that are intended to relieve pain as quickly as possible. While major symptoms are present, I suggest an "intensive care" approach to the exercises in which frequent repetition is the key to symptom relief.

The concept of repetition is one that I want to emphasize because I have given these recommendations to thousands of people over the years through both my chiropractic office as well as my websites and online instructional videos and the necessity of frequent repetition in the early stages of treatment is consistently missed. This is probably in part due to the way that exercises are typically presented by doctors and physical therapists.

The usual way that exercises for sciatica are presented is that the patient is either led through them in the doctor's or therapist's office in a supervised treatment session lasting 15 to 30 minutes with treatment sessions every day or every other day, or the patient is simply given a sheet of exercises and told to do them at home. At best, with these approaches, the patient does the exercises once or twice per day. For nerve compression sciatica related to a bulging disc, that usually is not enough to get lasting relief very quickly, so patients will often go for many weeks or months in pain with very slow improvement.

IMPORTANT NOTE*: What I have found is that during the early stages of treatment when symptoms are most severe, it works much better to do a minute or two of one or two effective exercises (such as the ones that follow in this chapter) several times every hour you are awake.

Let me repeat that – do a minute or two of effective exercises several times every **hour**! No, that's not a typo - I do mean several times an **hour**, not just a few times per **day**.

Now you may be thinking that's a lot - and it is, but most people don't need to keep up that frequency for very long. In most cases, a few days to a few weeks of multiple times per hour use of the exercises I'm about to present will drastically reduce the symptoms, and when that occurs, you can decrease the frequency of the exercises to just a few minutes each day for prevention (as we'll discuss in the chapter on prevention and rehabilitation).

The specific frequency of the exercises will vary somewhat according to the person. As a general rule, for individuals up to about 50 years of age, I suggest starting with doing each exercise for about a minute at a time at a frequency of 5 to 6 times every hour. For individuals over 50, I suggest starting with a frequency of about half that at 2 to 3 times every hour. This is because older individuals often have some degree of spinal arthritis, which can be temporarily irritated by the suggested exercises.

Many people will get some soreness in their backs or shoulders during the "intensive care" phase of the exercises. This is temporary, and can usually be eased with the use of ice as discussed earlier, and/or with massage. As long as the soreness is tolerable, I recommend continuing with the exercises at the recommended frequency, but you can always reduce the frequency of the exercise if needed.

One last point of clarification before I go into the exercises is the fact that from the standpoint of the health of nerves, numbness is worse than pain. While most people find numbness to be more comfortable than pain, numbness suggests greater and/or longer duration nerve compression than pain does. So, if you are starting out mostly with numbness and it is changing to pain, that is actually a good sign in most cases. On the other hand, if you start out with mostly pain and it is changing to numbness, that is often a bad sign and is an indication that you should change what you are doing and/or seek out professional treatment.

That being said, it is important to distinguish numbness, which is a lack of sensation, from "heaviness" or "tiredness" that sometimes occurs for a short time after severe pain goes away. If you're not sure which you are experiencing, lightly jab the effected area with a pin or needle (you don't need to break the skin) and compare the sensation to the same spot on the opposite side of your body or another spot that feels normal and compare them. If the pin/needle feels about the same on both spots, you are probably just experiencing heaviness resulting from muscles relaxing as the nerve irritation decreases.

Now let's begin with the pain relief exercises...

McKenzie Method Exercises

McKenzie method (named for physical therapist Robin McKenzie) are often associated with extension (backward bending) of the spine, but in reality they are about testing for, and then exercising in, positions and stretches that alleviate or produce "centralization" of symptoms.

Centralization means that the symptoms move closer to the spine. For example, if you have low back pain with sciatica (leg pain), centralization would be where the symptoms leave or lessen in the leg, even if the pain stays the same or gets worse in the buttocks or low back.

Centralization

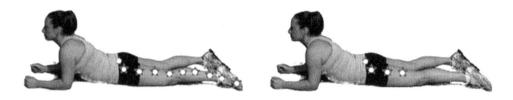

In the picture above, the concept of centralization is illustrated with the white dots representing the extension of symptoms down the leg. In the image on the left, the initial symptoms extend all the way to the foot, but as symptoms centralize the symptoms leave the foot and lower leg as shown in the image on the right.

Over time, in most cases the thigh, buttock, and low back pain will also improve in situations where initial centralization is achieved.

Because the vast majority of the time extension of the spine is beneficial in reducing or centralizing pain, McKenzie exercises are often called "McKenzie Extension Exercises", but true McKenzie Technique actually tests for the position(s) that are beneficial for an individual patient. So, although McKenzie exercises most often do involve extension of the spine, they can involve flexion (forward bending), and left or right side bending combined with extension or flexion – depending on what position reduces or centralizes symptoms. The following pictures illustrate the positions that should be tested and compared to determine the position that best centralizes symptoms:

Straight Extension

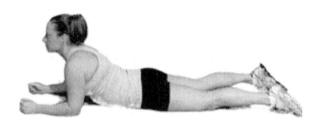

Extension With Left and Right Side Bending

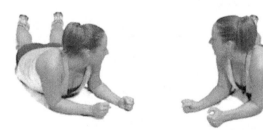

Flexion

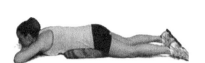 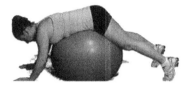

Note: For Flexion An Exercise Ball Works Best, But For Testing Purposes, A Pillow Or Stack Of Pillows Under The Abdomen Will Work. If Straight Flexion Is Helpful, Flexion Combined With Left And Right Side Bending Should Also Be Tested, But These Positions Are Rarely Used And Because They Can Dramatically Irritate Disc Related Symptoms These Positions Are Not Shown. Again, Flexion With Left and Right Side Bending Should Only Be Tested If Straight Flexion Is Helpful!

You will probably have some pain when you first move into a new position. After you get into each position, wait 30 seconds to a minute to see what happens with your symptoms. The thing to remember is that you are looking for a position that eases the symptoms the furthest away from the spine first.

For example, if you have sciatica all the way to the foot, a good position would be one that moves the pain out of the foot and calf, even if it intensifies pain in the buttocks or low back. If you only had sciatica in the buttock and thigh, a good position would be one that moves the pain out of the buttock and thigh, even if it gets worse in the low back.

If there is no clear "winner" as a position that best centralizes your symptoms, begin with using the straight extension position.

IMPORTANT NOTE*: Any position that makes the symptoms the furthest from the spine WORSE or causes symptoms to extend further from the spine should be avoided!

In other words, do NOT continue with any position that makes symptoms either more intense in the leg or extend further down the leg.

IMPORTANT NOTE*: If every position causes increased symptoms at the furthest point from the spine, and/or causes the symptoms to extend further down the leg from the spine, DO NOT perform any of the McKenzie exercises (in such cases, professional evaluation and

treatment is strongly recommended!).

Otherwise, keep testing different positions until you find the one that does the best job of alleviating the symptoms furthest from the spine. Once you find the position that works the best, hold that position for 1 to 2 minutes and then take a break for 30 seconds or so in a neutral position. Repeat the beneficial position frequently, as long as it continues to relieve the symptoms furthest from the spine.

Note, you will only be using the <u>one best position</u> that gives you the best centralization of symptoms.

You will not be using any of the other positions unless you reach a point where the chosen position no longer provides further centralization after 3 or more days of frequent use. If this occurs, re-test to see if a different position works better.

In most cases, one of the extension positions (straight extension, extension with left side-bending, or extension with right side-bending) will be the most effective. If that is the case with you, the following modification will usually enhance the benefits of the exercise:

Advanced McKenzie Extension Technique

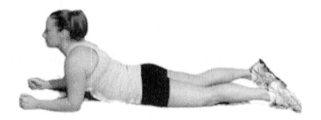

Begin as usual with the McKenzie exercise by propping yourself up on your elbows (and then bend left or right if one of these positions improved your results when using the basic McKenzie extension position).

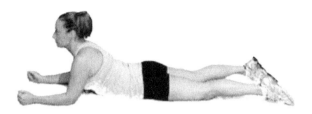

Next, shift your elbows forward an inch or two, as shown above.

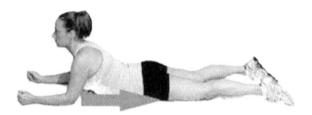

Finally, pull back with your arms, so that your upper body is pulled forward. Do not pull so hard that your lower body slides, but enough that you can feel a pull on the pelvis. This produces a mild traction on the low back and this traction combined with the spinal extension can be quite effective.

As an alternative to the lying flat on the floor version of spinal extension, you can achieve similar effects with spinal extension done on your hands and knees as shown in the next picture:

Modified McKenzie Extension Technique

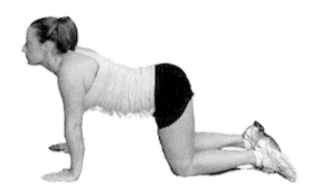

In the position above, simply allow the abdomen to hang down so that the spine curves towards the floor.

Exercises for Muscle Contraction Sciatica

If it appears that most of your symptoms are caused by nerve compression, I recommend that you skip the following exercises until such time as your symptoms have significantly improved (unless otherwise advised by a health care professional managing your care). Attempting to stretch muscles that are contracted due to nerve compression irritation will be of minimal benefit until the nerve compression has eased, and in some cases will actually irritate symptoms temporarily.

As previously discussed, repetition is key to getting the best results, so for the exercises that I'm about to discuss, I suggest holding the stretches for 30 seconds to a minute at a time and repeating them 5 to 6 times every hour you are awake. Age is less of a factor in the frequency recommendation than for the McKenzie exercises, but if you get too sore doing the stretches this much, you can decrease the frequency as needed.

One thing to keep in mind is that although you may only have symptoms on one side, it is a good idea to do the exercises that follow on both sides, as it is important to keep the muscles as balanced as possible. In addition, there is a neurological crossover effect that results in improved muscle flexibility on the opposite side of the one being stretched. So, stretching the asymptomatic side will actually help the symptomatic side to some degree. If you are having difficulty stretching the painful side, it may help to start by stretching the asymptomatic side first.

There are two muscles that commonly produce symptoms similar to sciatic nerve compression. Most often the muscle involved is the piriformis, but similar symptoms can be caused by the gluteus minimus muscle as well. Let's look at stretching exercises for these muscles:

Piriformis Stretching

The piriformis can be stretched in various ways in which the hip joint is flexed (bent forward) and rotated inward. The next image shows the method I recommend:

Basic Piriformis Stretch

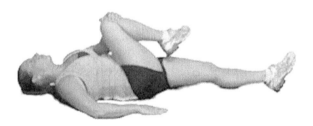

Piriformis stretch – pull the knee towards the opposite shoulder. Hold for 10 to 30 seconds and then switch and stretch the other leg. Repeat a few times with each leg and for best results do the stretch several times throughout the day.

Gluteus Minimus Stretching

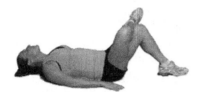 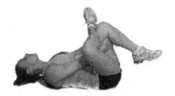

Begin by crossing the symptomatic leg's ankle over the other leg's knee as shown in the image on the left. then reach behind the knee and pull it towards your chest – you will likely feel soreness and/or pulling in the buttock area.

You may see the gluteus minimus stretch above referred to by some authors as a piriformis stretch. While any type of hip flexion will stretch the piriformis to some degree, the hip must be internally rotated to maximally stretch the piriformis. Flexion combined with external rotation maximally stretches the gluteus minimus muscle. You may need to stretch both muscles to get the best results, so if both feel tight, by all means stretch them both and don't be too concerned about which muscle it is!

That covers the exercises for pain relief. We'll be adding a few more exercises in the chapter on prevention, but for now, let's move on to other techniques for relieving pain.

Chapter 5: Massage And Positioning Techniques

Self-Massage

We just finished discussing stretching exercises for the piriformis and gluteus minimus muscles. In addition to stretching, it usually helps to massage these muscles as well. The following are self-massage techniques you can use, but professional massage therapy is quite beneficial as well.

As with stretching, if your symptoms appear to be mostly due to nerve irritation, I recommend that you skip this treatment measure until your symptoms are significantly better, because massage on a muscle that is contracted due to nerve compression irritation is of very temporary benefit and in some cases may temporarily increase symptoms.

Piriformis Massage

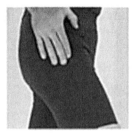 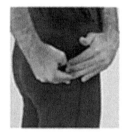 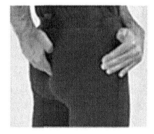

To find the piriformis muscle, begin by locating the outer part of the hip by placing the base of the palm of your hand on your waist and laying your fingers down the side of your pelvis. If you rotate your leg, you should feel the hip rotating under your fingers. Make note of where the hip is (you may want to keep one hand on it as shown above). Next, find the lower tip of the sacrum bone at the top of the "butt crack". The piriformis muscle runs from the outer edge of the sacrum to the hip, so one end will be just above your fingers on the sacrum and the other end will be just inside the fingers on your hip.

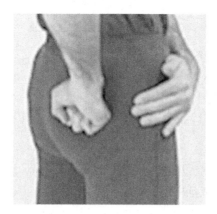

Feel for a tight and/or tender spot midway along the piriformis muscle (between the lower edge of the sacrum and hip joint) and massage with your knuckles or fingers in a circular motion.

Gluteus Minimus Massage

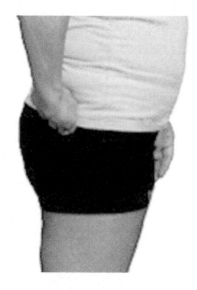

Feel for a tight and/or tender spot in the gluteus minimus (located in the middle of the upper buttock area 1 to 3 inches below your belt line) and massage with your knuckles or fingers in a circular motion.

Pelvic Repositioning

In many cases, with both nerve compression sciatica due to a bulging disc, and in muscle contraction sciatica, there is an underlying problem with the alignment/mobility of one or both of the sacroiliac joints, which are the joints where the pelvic bones meet the sacrum – the triangular bone at the base of the spine.

Depending on the severity of the problem, it may be possible to realign the sacroiliac joints using a simplified version of what chiropractors know as "Sacro-Occipital Technique" (SOT). This method uses wedges or pads placed under the pelvic bones.

In this simplified version, the pads will be used under the pelvis while you lie face down on a firm surface. It can be done on a bed, but bear in mind that the softer the surface you are on, the thicker the pads will need to be in order to reposition the pelvis.

I suggest using folded hand towels as the pads/pelvic supports as shown in the image below. You'll need to test the position of the pads to see which position works best, but because the majority of the time it works best with the upper pad on the left side and the lower pad on the right side, that's how I suggest you start and that is how the procedure is illustrated below.

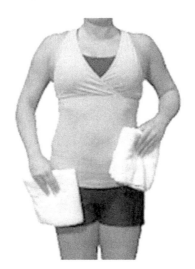

The relative position of the pelvic supports is shown above in the standing position so you can better tell where they go. The actual treatment position is shown in the next image below. You can use rolled up towels (make sure they

are the same size and rolled the same way), a pair of shoes, or even tennis balls to support the pelvis.

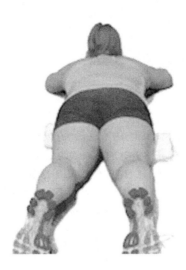

Here are the supports are shown in actual use. Begin with the supports placed with the upper one on the left side and the lower one on the right as shown above (this is the more commonly helpful positioning).

Lie on the supports for about 30 seconds. If there is no pain relief, try switching the supports to the opposite positioning (the higher support on the right and the lower support on the left). You may need to slide the supports up or down slightly to get them in the most comfortable position. Once you find a position that eases symptoms, you can stay on the pads for 3 to 5 minutes at a time and use this treatment method up to 3 or 4 times per day. Be careful not to overuse it, because over-correction of the sacroiliac joints can temporarily increase symptoms.

Enhancing Sitting Comfort

In some cases considerable symptom relief can be achieved while sitting by changing the alignment of the pelvis on the seat as shown in the next image.

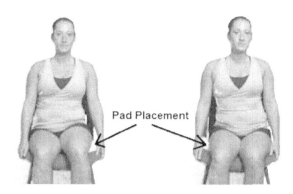

Place a folded towel or washcloth under one buttock and sit in a relaxed posture. Notice whether or not this feels more comfortable than without the lift. If the lift makes sitting less comfortable, move it to the other side and notice if that improves things. If not, try using different thicknesses of the lift and move it from side to side until you find a thickness and position that helps.

Chapter 6: Acupressure Techniques

Acupressure can be helpful for alleviating symptoms from both nerve compression and muscle contraction forms of sciatica.

Acupressure points can be stimulated by pressing / massaging with your fingers, "pulsing" them with the spring-loaded button of a ball-point pen (see picture below), or, if you happen to have a laser pointer available (a red laser with a 630 – 635 nm wavelength is recommended), you can direct the laser on the points.

Pen Button and Laser Methods Of Acupressure Stimulation

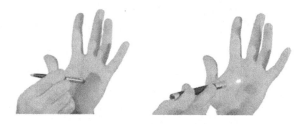

Regardless of the stimulation method, usually 2 to 3 minutes of stimulation per point is adequate to get results. Longer periods of stimulation are safe, and you can repeat the treatments as often as needed.

Don't let the location of the points confuse you - acupressure points may be nowhere near the site of pain, but they can still be very effective. You'll notice that some points are used for more than one site of pain. If you aren't sure if you're on the right spot, feel around in the general area where the point should be and you will usually find a tender spot – that is usually the point to treat.

It is usually most effective to treat the points on the side of the body where the pain is, so if you only have pain on one side, start with the points on that side, but it may be helpful to do the recommended points on both sides of the body.

Point GB34 For General Musculoskeletal Pain

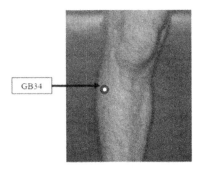

GB34 is a treatment point that can be used for any type of musculoskeletal pain. It is located about three finger widths below the kneecap on the outside area of the lower leg in a depression just in front of the top of the fibula bone. It is recommended that you begin with this point and then use the points that follow that correspond to your specific problem area(s).

Sciatica Points

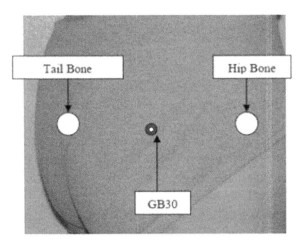

GB30 – located in the buttock between the hip and the tailbone.

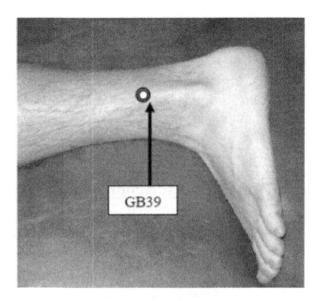

GB39 – located about 3 finger widths above the bone that sticks out on the outside of your ankle at the back edge of the bone.

Low Back Pain Points

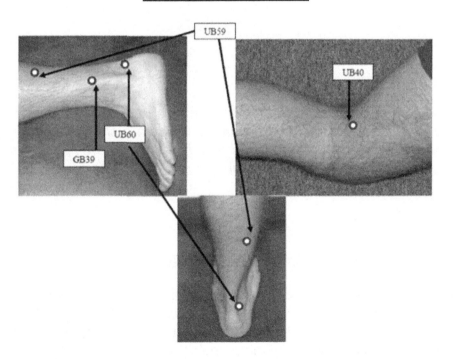

GB39 – can be used for low back pain as well as sciatica, as seen in the previous illustration, it is located about 3 finger widths above the bone that

sticks out on the outside of your ankle at the back edge of the bone. UB40 – located in the center of the back of the knee at the very lower end of the thigh bone. UB59 – located just to the outside of the Achilles tendon where it attaches to the lower calf muscle. UB60 – located just to the outside of the Achilles tendon about 1 finger width above the top of the heel bone.

Auriculotherapy (Ear Acupressure) Points

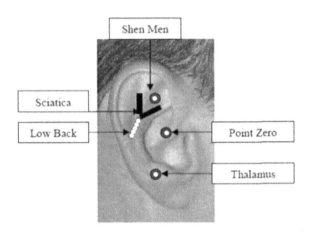

Shen men, point zero, and the thalamus point can be used for any pain, and the specific areas for the low back and sciatica are shown. Stimulation of these points is usually accomplished best by either the ball point pen button or laser pointer methods.

"Surround the Dragon"

Besides the specific points shown, there is a concept in acupressure called "Surround the Dragon" – which basically involves finding tender spots around the site of pain (search the edges of the painful area for points that are tender to touch), and then stimulating them (using any of the methods mentioned previously).

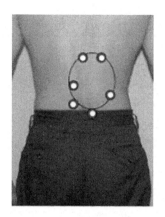

"Surround the Dragon" – if the circled area was where you felt pain, you would push with your fingers to find tender points around the border of the painful area and treat any points you find with either fingertip massage, pen-button stimulation, or laser stimulation.

Chapter 7: Supplements And Natural Remedies

There are numerous nutritional supplements, herbal products, and homeopathic remedies being promoted for the treatment of sciatica. All of these products probably work at least some of the time, whether by actual chemical therapeutic effect, or by means of the placebo effect.

When it comes to sciatica, the supplements and remedies that are most likely to have a therapeutic benefit are the ones that either have an anti-inflammatory effect, or correct some type of nutritional deficiency that results in nerve irritation and/or abnormal muscle contraction.

The list of possible supplements and remedies is incredibly long, so for the purposes of simplicity, the following recommendations has been limited to readily available supplements and remedies that have some amount of validation from scientific research and/or strong anecdotal evidence supporting their effectiveness and safety.

The suggestions that follow are in regards to particular vitamins, minerals, herbs, etc., not to particular brands. With regards to brand-name products, you should be aware that marketing hype often far exceeds actual results that can be expected with a given product.

Due to variability in the availability of certain products in different parts of the world, I do not make specific recommendations regarding brands. When it comes to choosing a brand, my recommendation is to look for a product that uses independent lab certification of the product as to its potency and purity. Optionally, it may be helpful to research the product on Amazon.com or other shopping website to look at user reviews of the product.

Natural Anti-Inflammatories

The anti-inflammatory supplements exert their effects by controlling the inflammatory response and thereby reducing swelling and pain. There are many such supplements, but among the most popular and best-documented by scientific research are: omega-3 fatty acids (EPA and DHA – mostly commonly from fish oil, but krill oil or walnut oil are also good sources), bromelain, hesperidin, quercetin, curcumin (turmeric), MSM, ginger, and aloe vera.

Homeopathic remedies for reducing pain and inflammation may also be useful, and there are many such remedies. For best results with homeopathy, I recommend consulting with a homeopathic physician to get the remedy that is best suited to your particular needs.

As with medications, different natural anti-inflammatories work better for one person than another. For the sake of simplicity, I recommend using either Omega-3 fatty acids (at a dose that provides approximately 1,000 mg of EPA per day), or a product with a combination of two or more of the other substances mentioned (follow package instructions for dosing recommendations). Ginger can also be eaten in various forms as opposed to being taken as a supplement - some people find candied crystallized ginger an effective and tasty anti-inflammatory.***

IMPORTANT NOTE*: If you are already taking either over-the-counter or prescription anti-inflammatories, or you are on blood-thinning drugs such as Coumadin (warfarin), it is strongly recommended that you consult with a pharmacist or licensed healthcare provider before starting any nutritional anti-inflammatories as there is a potential for dangerous interactions.

Correcting Nutrient Deficiencies

There are a few common deficiencies that can trigger sciatica and sciatica-like pain.

A deficiency of any or all of the B-vitamins can potentially trigger various nerve-related symptoms including sciatica. Of all of the B-vitamins, deficiency is probably most common in B-6 and B-12.

With regards to vitamin B-6 deficiency, the deficiency is sometimes due to a diminished ability of the body to convert the vitamin to the active form known as pyridoxal-5-phosphate (also known as P5P), as opposed to a lack of intake of B-6. For this reason, I suggest using a supplement that contains at least part of the B-6 in the pyridoxal-5-phosphate form. From a dosage standpoint, I suggest supplementing with 30 to 50 mg of pyridoxal-5-phosphate per day.

As with vitamin B-6 deficiency, vitamin B-12 deficiency is often due more to factors other than daily intake. Vitamin B-12 requires a substance produced by the body called "intrinsic factor" to be absorbed and utilized. Production of intrinsic factor will often be decreased in older individuals and people who have a history of alcohol abuse.

Because decreased intrinsic factor prevents the absorption of vitamin B-12, even supplementation with large oral doses of B-12 in solid form may not be sufficient to correct the deficiency. In such cases, deficiency can be corrected with either periodic injections of liquid vitamin B-12 by a licensed healthcare provider, or sublingual supplementation. Sublingual liquid vitamin B-12 is not as readily available as solid supplements and is not intended to be swallowed, but held in the mouth under the tongue for absorption directly into the blood stream through the mucous membranes of the mouth.

Before proceeding with either B-12 injections or sublingual supplementation, it is strongly advised that blood testing be done to establish whether or not there is actually a vitamin B-12 deficiency. Dosing depends on the concentration of the supplement used and the extent of the deficiency.

Another common deficiency that can produce sciatica-like symptoms is potassium deficiency. Potassium deficiency is most commonly seen in individuals who lose lot of fluid through perspiration, vomiting, or diarrhea, and in people with kidney disease. It can also occur as a side-effect of certain medications, such as those for high blood pressure - especially diuretics.

Mild potassium deficiency can usually be corrected safely by simply getting more potassium in the diet. Although bananas are the classic high-potassium food, many other foods are as good or better sources of potassium. These include melons, avocados, oranges, most green leafy vegetables, and blackstrap molasses. Potassium supplements are also available, but before taking high doses of potassium supplements, it is strongly recommended that blood testing be performed to measure potassium levels - too much potassium can be dangerous!

One other deficiency that can create sciatica-like symptoms, although usually as a part of all-over body pain, is Coenzyme Q-10 (or CoQ10 for short). This deficiency is very frequently the result of a side-effect of cholesterol-lowering drugs. There are two options in handling the deficiency. The first is to supplement with coenzyme Q-10 at a suggested starting dose of 200 mg per day. If this relieves symptoms, the dosage can usually be reduced to 50 to 100 mg per day for maintenance. If there is no benefit, and symptoms do seem to be related to cholesterol-lowering medication, it is recommended that the issue be discussed with your physician and perhaps you can switch to a different medication or discuss alternatives to allow you to get off of the medication altogether.

Although coenzyme Q-10 is generally safe and well-tolerated, it does have the potential to thin the blood, and therefore if you are on aspirin therapy or stronger anticoagulant medication (such as Coumadin), you should consult your doctor or pharmacist before starting coenzyme Q-10.

Finally, although not technically a deficiency, some diabetics will experience symptoms in the legs that can be mistaken for sciatica that are related to nerve damage caused by decreased circulation. These symptoms can sometimes be helped by supplementation with alpha-lipoic acid, which is a strong anti-oxidant. For long-term use, a daily dosage of about 50 mg per day is recommended. Larger doses are sometimes recommended for short-term use, but should only be done under the supervision of a health care professional.

Chapter 8: Releasing Emotional Pain Triggers

It is not uncommon for physical pain and other symptoms to be triggered or increased by emotional factors. There are many methods for handling negative emotional states, but one of the simplest methods I've found that is well-suited to self-treatment is called Emotional Freedom Technique, or EFT for short.

Emotional Freedom Technique is most often used as a means of handling negative emotions and as a means of habit control, but it can be very helpful in dealing with pain as well. EFT combines acupressure with verbal affirmations to change your emotional state. I will summarize the basic procedure here and most people will do quite well just using the basics, but you can also download a free full-length manual on this method, as well as get information on seminars and advanced instruction by going to www.EFTuniverse.com.

As I said, Emotional Freedom Technique uses acupressure stimulation along with verbal affirmations to change the "emotional charge" or intensity of a physical pain, craving, habit, phobia, or traumatic event. The starting point of the procedure is to identify whatever it is you want to change, and then verbalize it in the form of a self-accepting affirmation while tapping a series of points.

For example, let's say you are experiencing sciatica. For the purposes of doing Emotional Freedom Technique, you will always use the structure of "Even though I [insert undesirable symptom, behavior, or emotion here], I deeply and completely accept myself." So, using the example of sciatica, you would say, "Even though I am having sciatica, I deeply and completely accept myself."

In the case of pain and other symptoms, you may be able to associate a certain emotional event or stressful situation to the onset or increase of the symptoms. In fact, sometimes simply noticing the words we use can clue us in on emotional issues that may be triggering physical symptoms.

Even though most cases of sciatica are related to objective disc injuries, you might be surprised at how much of a role emotional issues can play. For instance, if you are unhappy at work and think your boss is a "pain in the butt", you may very well experience increased physical sciatica pain in the buttock area when you have to deal with your boss.

Diminishing the "charge" of underlying emotional issues can bring a surprising amount of pain relief in some cases. Although other techniques for using affirmations may recommend phrasing your affirmations in terms of the way you want things to be (such as, "I feel healthy and pain-free!"), this is not how they are used with Emotional Freedom Technique. So, as another example, let's say that you recognize that emotional issues from dealing with your boss may be participating in your physical symptoms, you could use the affirmation, "Even though I feel like my boss is a pain in the butt, I deeply and completely accept myself."

Whatever the affirmation for your specific issue, you repeat it out loud as you tap a series of acupressure points. The sequence and location of the points is shown on the next page. For each point, you'll tap it 7 or 8 times with a finger tip as you repeat the affirmation out loud. Tap the points in the number sequence shown, starting at point 1 above the eye and working through to point 13 (if you download the full manual from the Emotional Freedom Technique website, you'll see that I have added one finger point – this point is optional and I have included it only because it is easier to just do all of the fingers than try to remember which one you don't need to do).

It usually does not matter whether you do points on the left or right side of the body, but I find it usually works better to stick to one side, rather than doing some points on the left and some on the right. You may find that tapping the points on the side of pain works the best.

Points for Emotional Freedom Technique

(The points are indicated as dots on the pictures that follow the list.)

1. Over Eye
2. Outside Corner Of Eye
3. Under Eye
4. Between Nose And Upper Lip
5. Between Lower Lip And Chin
6. Just Below Where Collar Bone Joins Breastbone
7. Center Of Arm Pit
8. Outer Edge Of Base Of Thumb Nail
9. Outer Edge (Thumb Side) Of Base Of Index Finger Nail
10. Outer Edge (Thumb Side) Of Base Of Middle Finger Nail
11. Outer Edge (Thumb Side) Of Base Of Ring Finger Nail
12. Outer Edge (Thumb Side) Of Base Of Little ("Pinky") Finger Nail

42 • Sciatica Exercises & Home Treatment

13. "Karate Chop" Point On Outer Edge of Hand Midway Between Little Finger and Wrist

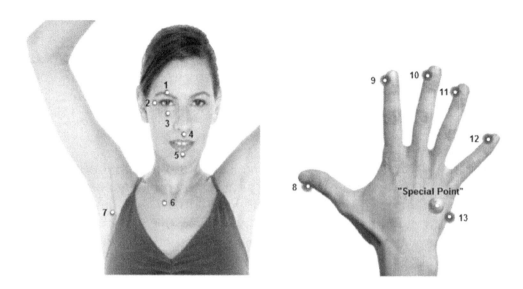

After you have tapped on the series of points while repeating the affirmation ("Even though I [insert undesirable symptom, behavior, or emotion here], I deeply and completely accept myself."), the next step is to activate various brain centers while tapping on what I'll call the "special point" point on the back of the hand, on a line directly between the ring finger and little finger, midway between the base of the fingers and the wrist (as shown on the hand image in the picture above).

As you tap on the "special point", you'll go through a series of steps as follows:

1. Open your eyes.
2. Close your eyes.
3. Open your eyes and, without moving your head, look down and left with your eyes.
4. Open your eyes and, without moving your head, look down and right with your eyes.
5. Circle ("roll") your eyes clockwise.
6. Circle ("roll") your eyes counter-clockwise.
7. Hum a tune for a few seconds (any familiar tune will work, such as the "Happy Birthday" song).
8. Count out loud from one to five ("one, two, three, four, five").
9. Hum a tune again for a few seconds.

Once you have completed these procedures while tapping the "special point", there's one more step. Once again, you will tap 7 or 8 times on each of the 13 points done in the initial step, this time while repeating just the word or phrase that describes the undesirable symptom, habit, behavior, or emotion. For example, if your affirmation in the first step of the procedure was, "Even though I have sciatica, I deeply and completely accept myself," this time through you will repeat just the word, "sciatica" while you tap the points.

After one time through the entire procedure, most people will have significant improvement in the symptoms, habit, behavior, or emotion they wish to change. If there is no improvement, you may want to think about underlying issues that are related to the problem you wish to address. For example, if your pain started shortly after a major fight with your wife about your finances, you might switch from a symptom-focused affirmation like "Even though I have sciatica..." to "Even though I disagree with my wife about our finances...".

If there is some, but not 100% improvement, the procedure can be repeated with a variation in the affirmation used in the initial step and the phrase used in the final step. For repeats of the procedure, there is an acknowledgment of the prior issue being somewhat improved.

For example, if the first time through the procedure your affirmation was, "Even though I have sciatica, I deeply and completely accept myself.", your affirmation for the first step each time you repeat the procedure will be, "Even though I **still have some remaining sciatica**, I deeply and completely accept myself.". And for the final step of the procedure for the repeats, the phrase would change from "sciatica" to "remaining sciatica". Otherwise, the procedure for repeats is the same as when you do it the first time for a given issue.

In some cases, you may need to get more specific with your affirmation to help with the problem you are experiencing. For instance, if you are having problems with left buttock pain, it may be more effective to say, "Even though I have pain in my left buttock..." than to say "Even though I have sciatica...". The more specific you can be and the more you can deal with any possible emotional triggers for your pain, the more effective EFT will be.

Chapter 9: Prevention Of Sciatica

The Importance of Prevention

It is important to understand that in most cases the underlying causes of sciatica (especially bulging discs) typically remain to varying degrees long after the symptoms are gone. It usually only takes a tiny reduction in disc bulging and/or a minor reduction in inflammatory swelling to reduce or eliminate symptoms, but it also only takes a small increase in disc bulging or inflammation to cause the symptoms to return. Even when the symptoms are completely gone, the underlying bulging disc is usually far from totally healed and will typically cause trouble again at some point in the future if it is not properly managed.

In addition, while people are sometimes surprised by a return of symptoms after an extended period of feeling good, it is only reasonable to expect that the same activities, postures, and lifestyle choices that may have led to the initial episode of sciatica could cause subsequent episodes. This is true with both disc-related nerve compression sciatica as well as sciatica-like symptoms from the piriformis and/or gluteus minimus muscles.

With this in mind, I strongly encourage people to think in terms of managing sciatica rather than curing it. While it would be nice if there was a once and for all cure, the reality is that a certain amount of ongoing preventive care is necessary to keep the symptoms from returning and getting worse over time.

Even in many cases where the patient has undergone surgical treatment, the potential for sciatica to return is high if the patient does not take steps to prevent future problems. While complete discectomy (removal of a disc) guarantees that the patient will never have symptoms from that disc again, such procedures shift mechanical stresses to other discs and spinal structures which often do become damaged and produce symptoms months or years later. Judging from my experiences with post-surgical cases, many surgeons fail to adequately explain this to their patients, so these patients are unaware of the need for ongoing preventive measures.

The good news is that effective prevention is usually pretty easy to manage. While doctors and physical therapists will sometimes discharge patients with a long list of home exercises and other preventive treatments, in my experience, very few patients will continue to spend 20 to 30 minutes or more every day performing a long list of exercises, especially when they are no longer in pain. Fortunately, effective prevention does not require a lot of time nor a complicated list of exercises. As with getting initial symptom relief, doing a few highly effective exercises typically works better in the long run than trying to keep up with many different exercises.

By combining a few minutes of preventive exercise each day with awareness and avoidance of activities and postures that tend to cause the development of sciatica, most people are able to stay symptom free at least most of the time.

So, let's discuss the key points to preventing sciatica and other low back conditions.

Back Safe Posture and Lifting

While people often assume that pain as severe as sciatica must be caused by a major trauma, poor sitting posture (particularly when you sit frequently and/or for long periods of time) is actually one of the most common issues that can lead to bulging discs that produce back pain and sciatica.

Poor Sitting Posture

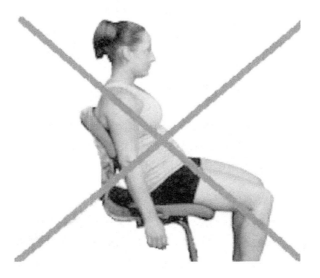

Sitting with the lower back unsupported places considerable stress on the back portion of the spinal discs and can cause or worsen disc bulges associated with sciatica and back pain.

Prolonged sitting (sitting for more than an hour at a time) is potentially harmful to the back when done on a daily or frequent basis under even the best of conditions, but maintaining good sitting posture as shown below will minimize the damaging effects.

Good Sitting Posture

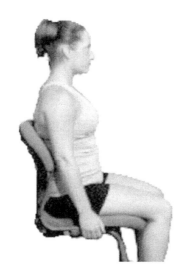

Sitting with the lower back supported. Even in the best of situations though, prolonged sitting is hard on the lower back, so getting up and moving around for at least a minute or two every half hour or so is highly recommended.

Sleep Position

While sleep position can be difficult to control (many people wind up in some very contorted positions while sleeping), it is worth the time to try to get in the habit of sleeping in a "back-friendly" position.

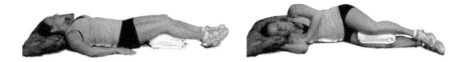

For most people with back pain and sciatica, the best sleep positions are lying on the back with a pillow or folded towel under the legs, or lying on the side with a pillow or folded towel between the legs as shown above.

Bending and Lifting

Improper bending and lifting is another common way that people cause injuries to their backs that result in back pain and sciatica. While most people have heard the advice to "lift with your legs", they may not be aware of the real goal which is to keep the lumbar spine from bending forward when standing or sitting.

In addition to avoiding weight-bearing forward bending of the lumbar spine, it is also important to minimize torque (twisting) and leverage on the spine (from loads held far out in front of the body) when lifting and carrying anything heavy.

The following are the most common bending and lifting positions to avoid:

Poor Bending, Lifting, and Carrying

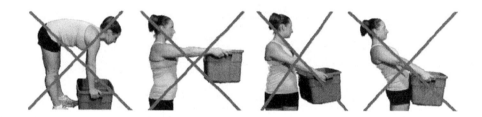

Avoid bending forward at the waist with your legs straight, carrying heavy objects away from your body, twisting with a heavy object, and/or hyper-extending your back to lift something that is really too heavy for you.

Attempting to lift something that is too heavy for you is unsafe no matter how good your lifting technique is, but good lifting form will greatly minimize the risk of injury when bending and lifting and should be used even with very light weights, since your own body weight is sufficient to cause injury with the unsafe bending and lifting techniques just discussed.

Safer Bending, Lifting, and Carrying

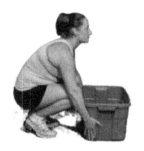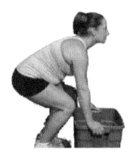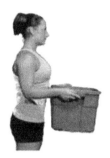

Bend your legs and keep your head up when lifting. If you have trouble bending your knees, stick your butt out and keep your back as straight as possible to allow you to lift safely without bending your knees as much (as shown in the middle picture above). Try to carry heavy objects close to your body.

Preventive Exercises

The same exercises you used for symptom relief earlier should be continued on a preventive basis as well, just at a reduced frequency from what you did during the "intensive care" phase.

If your symptoms appeared to be related to a bulging disc and you got relief with one of the McKenzie exercise positions, you should continue using that exercise for a minute or so at a time, a few times each day. If you were using one of the side-bending positions (extension with left or right side-bending or flexion with left or right side-bending) for pain relief, I recommend you also do the corresponding straight position (extension or flexion) a few times per day once you are in the prevention stage.

If you had a muscular component and benefitted from stretching of the piriformis and/or gluteus minimus, it is recommended that you continue to use those stretches for 30 seconds to a minute at a time, a few times on both sides every day once you reach the prevention stage.

In addition to the exercises you found most helpful for symptom relief, I suggest you add a couple of additional exercises that address the most common weaknesses and imbalances that contribute to the development of back pain and sciatica. Because of the huge variation in the people who are likely to use this book, the exercises I'm about to present are designed to be appropriate for a wide range of ages and levels of physical conditioning.

Young, fit individuals may find these exercises too easy. In that case, it is certainly acceptable to perform more demanding exercises, but it is suggested that you check with a healthcare provider familiar with your condition first to be sure that your choice of exercises is safe and appropriate.

The Pelvic Tilt

Basic Version

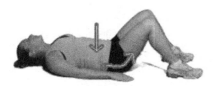 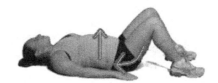

The Basic Pelvic Tilt: Begin by lying on your back on a firm surface with your knees bent. In this position, there should be some space between your low back and the surface you are lying on (you should be able to slide your hand part way under your low back). Contract your abdominal muscles and tilt your pelvis so that you press your low back down towards the surface and take out the space between the back and the surface. Hold for about 10 seconds. Relax and allow the space to return under your back, then tilt your pelvis the opposite direction and increase the space under the low back for a few moments. Relax again to the starting position.

Repeat the full cycle frequently to get used to the movement, as you will be doing a similar movement for the advanced (standing up) version and it is easier to get the feel for the exercise when lying down. When you are comfortable with this version of the exercise and can feel the movement in the back and the pelvis when you do it, you can move on to the advanced exercise shown next.

Advanced Version

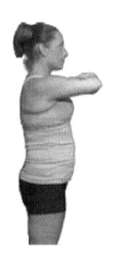 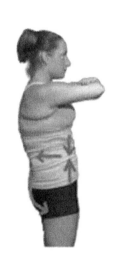 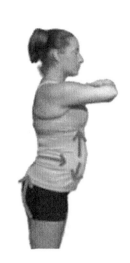

The Advanced Pelvic Tilt: Begin by standing in a relaxed posture. Contract your abdominal muscles, pulling them inward and tilt your pelvis so that it rotates as shown by the arrows. Hold for about 10 seconds and then relax. Continue on by further relaxing the abdominal muscles, arching the low back slightly and tilting your pelvis as shown. The movement is strictly in the pelvis and low back – the knees do not bend. Repeat 10 to 15 times in both directions. If possible, perform this exercise a few times per day, and as frequently as possible if you must sit a lot.

The Slouch and Arch

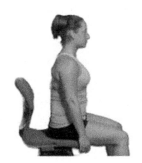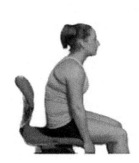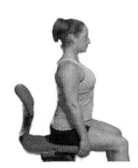

The Slouch and Arch: Begin by sitting on a chair or firm surface, with your feet flat on the floor. If you are in a chair, slide forward slightly so that there are a few inches between your back and the back of the chair. Allow yourself to slouch down, rounding your lower back as shown. Slowly sit up very straight and hold this position for 10 seconds. Then slowly allow yourself to slouch again and when you reach the slouched position, start to sit up straight again, in a slow, controlled movement. Note that the movement of the slouch and arch exercise is up and down, not leaning forward and backward. Repeat the process, alternating between the slouch and arch positions, pausing only for a moment in the slouch position and holding the arch position for about 10 seconds each time. 20 to 25 repetitions per session is suggested and one to three sessions per day is usually sufficient.

Preventive Exercise Summary

My recommendation for a sciatica prevention exercise routine consists of:

1. The McKenzie exercise in the position you used for pain relief plus the corresponding straight position if you were using one of the side-bending positions. If your problem was primarily muscular and you did not use the McKenzie exercise for pain relief, it is still advisable to use the straight extension position for prevention unless it causes pain or you have been directed to avoid spinal extension by a health care provider. I suggest holding the position for approximately one minute each time and do 2 to 4 repetitions.

2. The piriformis and/or gluteus minimus stretch (if your pain was mostly

muscular). You may skip this exercise if you did not find it useful for pain relief, but it is also fine to do it if you wish to. I suggest stretching each side for 30 seconds at a time and do 2 to 4 repetitions.

3. The advanced pelvic tilt (or more advanced abdominal "core" exercises) at least 10 to 15 repetitions per set, 2 to 4 sets.

4. The slouch and arch 20 to 25 repetitions per set, 2 to 4 sets.

It is strongly recommended that the above routine be done at least once per day. In most cases the exercises can be completed within 10 to 12 minutes. I suggest setting aside a specific time of day to do them and make them part of your daily routine so that you do them consistently.

One other preventive exercise recommendation I have is walking. A 10 to 20 minute walk every day or every other day is not only good for your back, it is also beneficial for relieving stress and general health and wellness. I suggest walking outside when practical (when weather and air quality permits), but walking on a treadmill or elliptical machine, or simply walking inside your home or office is fine as well.

Chapter 10: When To See A Doctor

While this book is dedicated to self-treatment methods, there are times when professional evaluation and treatment is necessary. In most situations, there is no harm in "toughing it out" and allowing time for the body to heal itself. There are some warning signs you need to be aware of though, that indicate the development of serious problems that can result in permanent disability if not cared for promptly.

Cauda Equina Syndrome

Cauda equina syndrome is a condition in which severe nerve compression is present and it requires fast medical attention in order to avoid permanent nerve damage. The symptoms of cauda equina syndrome may include the loss of bladder and/or bowel control, severe weakness in one or both legs, and what is known as "saddle anaesthesia" - the loss of sensation in the inner thighs and lower buttock and pelvic area (basically the area that would contact a saddle when horseback riding).

If you develop these symptoms, it is strongly recommended that you get immediate medical attention to evaluate the cause and correct the situation as quickly as possible.

Failure to Improve Within 2 to 3 Weeks

While severe cases can take several weeks to get significant improvement, and even mild to moderate cases may take several weeks to fully recover, a good rule of thumb is to look for overall improvement over any 2 to 3 week period of time. Now, most people experience at least a few ups and downs over the course of their recovery, but the trend over a period of a few weeks should be towards improvement. If you are no better off after 2 to 3 weeks of self-treatment, I strongly recommend that you see a doctor if you have not already.

If you have already seen a doctor and you are not improving, I recommend asking your doctor to explain any reasons that may be delaying your recovery and to give you an estimate of how long he or she expects it to take for you to begin improving. If your doctor doesn't seem willing or able to set any expectations for you, a second opinion is probably in order.

Pain Becoming Numbness

As mentioned previously, although more tolerable for most people, from a neurological perspective numbness is worse than pain. Numbness often indicates a greater severity and/or duration of nerve compression and is potentially a sign of decreasing nerve function and possible nerve damage. The longer numbness is present, the more likely that permanent nerve damage will occur and full recovery will not be possible.

Again, it is important to distinguish between true numbness (loss of sensation) and the "dull" or "heavy" sensation that sometimes occurs after intense pain is suddenly relieved. If you aren't sure which you are experiencing, lightly stick the area with a pin or needle (don't break the skin!) and compare the sensation of that to the same area on the other side of the body, or in a nearby spot that feels normal to you. If the pin/needle stick feels significantly less intense on the symptomatic area, you are likely having true numbness and professional care is recommended.

Conclusion

While sciatica and sciatica-like symptoms can be quite painful and scary to go through, the good news is that the vast majority of cases can be effectively managed with the self-treatment methods that have been presented. Even in more severe cases for which professional treatment is necessary, symptoms can usually be brought under control and long-term disability can be avoided.

For additional information, including Dr. Best's member resources that include video tutorials of the self-treatment methods presented in this book, or to send questions to Dr. Best, readers are invited to visit:

www.SciaticaTreatmentAtHome.com

About The Author

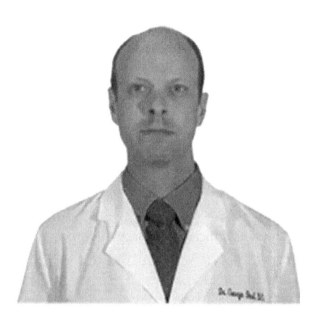

Dr. George F. Best, D.C. is a 1991 Summa Cum Laude graduate of Parker University (formerly Parker College Of Chiropractic) in Dallas, Texas. Dr. Best was valedictorian of his chiropractic school class and was the 1991 recipient of the *W. Karl Parker Award for Scholastic Excellence*. He has been in private practice in San Antonio, Texas since 1992.

In addition to treating numerous sciatica patients in his chiropractic practice, Dr. Best has provided consulting to sciatica sufferers and health care providers from all over the world through his websites SciaticaSelfCare.com and SciaticaTreatmentAtHome.com, and through his health-related YouTube channel (http://www.youtube.com/user/DrGeorgeBest).

Review And Connect

If you have found this book helpful, please consider posting a review at your favorite book retailer website or any of your preferred book review websites.

Dr. George Best may be contacted via the contact forms on his websites SciaticaSelfCare.com and SciaticaTreatmentAtHome.com.

Made in the USA
Coppell, TX
02 July 2021